Birkam Hot Yoga And Moksha Hot Yoga For Beginners

The Inner Workings Of Bikram And Moksha Hot Yoga

By: Amy Gilchrist

ISBN-13: 978-1491035306

TABLE OF CONTENTS

PUBLISHERS NOTES

Disclaimer

This publication is intended to provide helpful and informative material. It is not intended to diagnose, treat, cure, or prevent any health problem or condition, nor is intended to replace the advice of a physician. No action should be taken solely on the contents of this book. Always consult your physician or qualified health-care professional on any matters regarding your health and before adopting any suggestions in this book or drawing inferences from it.

The author and publisher specifically disclaim all responsibility for any liability, loss or risk, personal or otherwise, which is incurred as a consequence, directly or indirectly, from the use or application of any contents of this book.

Any and all product names referenced within this book are the trademarks of their respective owners. None of these owners have sponsored, authorized, endorsed, or approved this book.

Always read all information provided by the manufacturers' product labels before using their products. The author and publisher

© **2013**

Manufactured in the United States of America

DEDICATION

This book is dedicated to those who seek inner peace.

DEFINITION

Bikram yoga is a type of Hatha yoga created by Bikram Choudhury. This newer style of yoga was developed in recent years, but the art of yoga actually dates back to ancient times. The mind-body connection established while practicing Bikram yoga makes it beneficial for your total well-being. Including Bikram yoga in your weight loss and fitness plan is an effective way to lose weight, get fit and get rid of belly fat in the process.

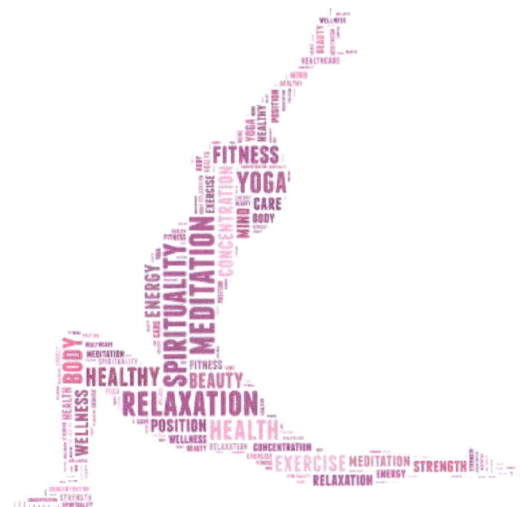

CHAPTER 1- WHAT YOU NEED TO KNOW ABOUT BIKRAM YOGA

Bikram yoga, also known as hot yoga, is an increasingly popular form of yoga in which practitioners move through traditional yoga poses in a room ideally heated to over one-hundred degrees. The heat of the room not only makes the workout more strenuous, thus burning more calories, but it also causes the body to sweat out impurities. If you have been considering dropping in on a hot yoga class to see what it's all about, here are a few tips and inside information to make your first experience successful and enjoyable.

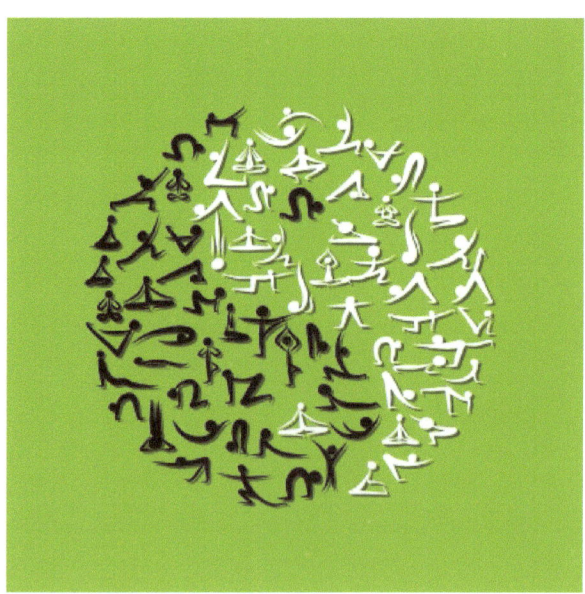

Gym Workouts are not the Same as Yoga Workouts

Even if you are in excellent shape and spend hours at the gym, you need to realize that yoga utilizes an entirely different set of muscles. Even if you practice yoga in a cooler room, chances are you will experience some muscle soreness the day after, and possibly even the day of. Just like starting any other workout, your muscles will have to adjust, so don't expect to be a rock star at it from day one.

Bring a Towel or Two

Have you ever been out on a hot, humid day and not sweat at least a little bit? Probably not. Now imagine doing an intense workout in that same heat, and there you have Bikram yoga. Everyone sweats, and it can make it difficult to do the positions when you don't have a towel to wipe sweat off your hands and knees. If possible, bring a second towel to lay over your mat since dripping sweat could make your mat slippery.

Wear Your Contacts

For anyone who needs vision correction, it's best to stick with contacts during Bikram yoga. Your eyeglasses will likely slide down your nose, and you'll be too busy pushing them back up to hold proper poses. This might not be a problem for practitioners who know the poses, but beginners will need to see the instructor to mimic the poses. If you can't wear contacts and you absolutely need some form of vision correction, be sure to bring an adjustable eyeglass lanyard.

Eat at Least an Hour (or Two!) Before Class

It's important to eat before a workout to have energy, but because of the hot, strenuous conditions of Bikram yoga, you should never eat directly before class. A light, balanced meal about two hours before class is best because the heat of the room along with the high activity level can make you feel nauseous, even without a stomach full of food to digest. Don't stick to just one type of food either. A belly full of carbs will take longer to digest than a banana and yogurt. If you've eaten a heavy meal that day, it's best to wait several hours before attending class. And early morning classes might do best without any food at all.

Dizzy? Take a Break

Bikram yoga is notorious for making its practitioners feel a little nauseous and dizzy from the combination of heat and physical exertion. Expect this feeling, but don't push yourself beyond your limits. If you are new to the practice or feel like you're pushing too hard, go to child's pose (a yoga pose in which you tuck your knees under your body and lay face down on the floor) until you feel ready for more. Your instructor would rather you miss a few poses than make yourself sick.

Bikram yoga isn't for everyone, but it can be an extremely rewarding practice, both physically and mentally. As with any workout, be sure to bring lots of water to replenish what you sweat out. If you know what to expect before you practice, you will be better prepared, and more likely to succeed.

CHAPTER 2- OVERVIEW OF POWER YOGA

Power yoga is an energetic and physically intense approach to yoga. Whether you try power yoga training in a Baron Baptiste studio or at your local gym, you should expect to sweat and feel challenged. Power yoga can work as a catch-all term to describe many intermediate or advanced yoga classes, or sometimes, to refer to yoga practiced in a hot room.

Characteristics

Linking poses with the breath, or vinyasa, is a commonly used tool in power yoga classes. According to the Ashtanga Yoga Institute, vinyasa produces sweat, which in turn, cleanses the body. Instructors may structure an entire power yoga class around vinyasa, or teach challenging poses, which students hold for long periods of time. A class might include arm balance poses such as crow or eight angle pose or sequences, which start from a mild pose, then build up to a complex variation. Some studios use heat. For example, students practice Bikram yoga in a room set at 105 degrees Fahrenheit.

Power Yoga Schools

Despite the challenging nature of power yoga classes, most yoga schools that offer the format are welcoming to beginners. The Bikram's Yoga College of India encourages a daily practice of their style, even for brand new students. Although power yoga classes often support the idea of bringing the body and mind to challenging places, they tend to balance that with the idea of Ahimsa, or non-violence. Students should avoid contraindicated poses for specific medical conditions or those which cause pain. When in doubt, start out with beginner or gentle yoga classes.

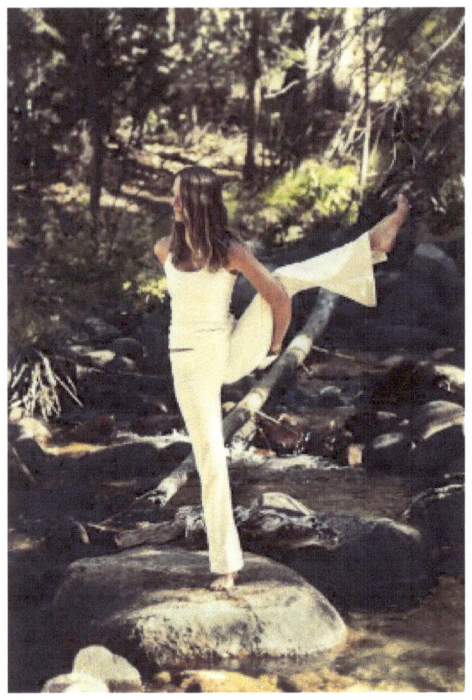

Effects

Power yoga has a reputation among yoga students for helping with weight management. According to the Bikram Yoga Portsmouth center, this style of power yoga burns up to 1,200 calories in a 90 minute session. Bikram's Yoga College of India and the Ashtanga Yoga Institute purport that their yoga styles purify the body and heal, or alleviate, many ailments. The discipline which power yoga demands of the mind when it focuses on holding yoga poses also prepares students for meditation and a deeper spiritual life.

Teacher Training

Power yoga teacher training all depends on the particular style of yoga on which you want to focus. You can take certifications for specific styles of power yoga such as Ashtanga or Baptiste. Other yoga schools, like Bryan Kest's Power Yoga, have close ties to the roots of Ashtanga, but have their own twists to the style. Yoga teacher training programs often require immersions of one week or longer. The most important preparation for any power yoga training program is a personal, daily practice of yoga.

Chapter 3- Choosing the Right Yoga Classes

For several weeks, Anna had been bugging her mother, Cathy, to try the yoga class she had been taking. Finally, Cathy went. At the end of the class, Cathy told her daughter that yoga was not for her; she did not like it, and would not go again. A year later a friend of Cathy's invited her to her yoga class and after much protestation, Cathy finally gave in and went. She went just to get her friend off her back. This time when the class ended Cathy felt yoga was just the thing she needed and readily signed up for a series of classes. What was it that made Cathy hate yoga the first time and love it the second time?

For Cathy, there were differences between the classes: The styles of yoga taught were not the same, and the teachers' demeanors were dissimilar, resulting in Cathy's expectations being met in the second class. In the first yoga class Cathy attended, the yoga was physically demanding; she thought the teacher was almost militaristic. Especially, after the teacher told Cathy that she would have her flexible and in shape in 3 months. This was not the perception Cathy had about yoga. She thought the class would move slower and the poses would be gentle. In the second class, that is what she found. Choosing a yoga class and teacher that is a good fit makes all the difference in the experience a person comes away with and whether they stay with yoga.

With over 20 styles of yoga and with estimates of over 50,000 teachers nationwide, choosing a class that is right for you can be daunting. However, having some knowledge about what to look for will give you the confidence to seek out the yoga class that is right for you.

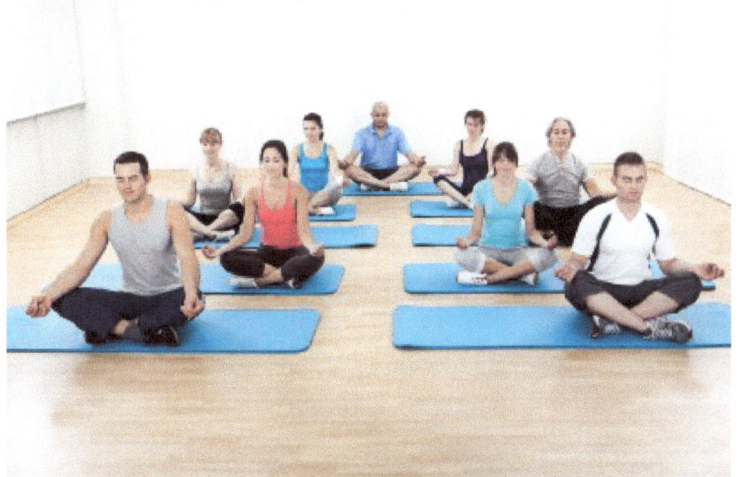

Safety First

The right fit with a yoga teacher begins with safety. It is one thing to come away with a little soreness from stretching tight muscles, and another thing to leave class with a dislocated knee cap because the knee was twisted while in Warrior II. Sore muscles should feel better after a few days; a kneecap out of alignment could have a long term effect on the body. Yoga like any other physical exercise program requires you to be responsible for what your body can and cannot do. However, you want to make sure that the class has a framework for you to be safe within.

In the yoga community, there are 2 schools of thought regarding regulating teachers. One side believes that given the proliferation of the yoga industry, there needs to be uniformity and standards by which teachers are certified. The other side of this discussion believes that regulating the teaching of yoga conflicts with the different traditions and nature of the discipline. They also believe that licensing or registering does not guarantee a professional is competent.

Yoga, teachers are not regulated or licensed by any state. However, there are organizations like Yoga Alliance that have set standards for teachers registered with them. Yoga Alliance and other registering organizations usually require that yoga teachers have a minimum of 200 hours of yoga instruction that not only covers postures, but also covers basic body anatomy, nutrition, philosophy, and ethical behavior. Yoga Alliance also regulates schools that teach yoga.

To be sure, there are excellent yoga teachers who are not registered. However, you do not want a teacher who has read a book, or who has taken a few classes and now thinks she can teach yoga. So, to ensure that you have a somewhat competent teacher ask them were they were trained and how much training they have had. If they were self-taught, you may want to investigate further into their knowledge of yoga.

As mentioned before, credentials do not always translate into having practical knowledge. So, take a class or two and observe the teacher. Here are some things to notice: Is she aware of proper body alignment? While demonstrating a pose or when students are practicing, does she talk about alignment; does she assist students with proper alignment? (There are some styles of yoga where the teachers do not do physical assists or walk among the students. They verbally instruct and direct students.)

Does she offer suggestions for other ways to do a pose, or use props for those students who are physically challenged with a posture? Is she pushing students to go beyond what their bodies are capable of doing? This observation is most noticeable in how she treats a student who is not in full extension of a posture. Is she telling you what your body can do instead of encouraging you to listen to your own body and go at your own pace? Is the teacher compassionate? How does she frame the study of yoga?

Beware of the teacher who construes proper alignment to mean a "perfect posture." There is no perfect posture or look in yoga. Given that each person's body is unique, there can be no universal form to a yoga position. You want a teacher that understands this and works with you where you are.

Contrary to what is happening in a lot of yoga classes, yoga is not a competitive sport. That includes being competitive with yourself. When competition enters the yoga class, injuries are bound to happen. You want a teacher to remind you that yoga is not a competitive exercise and that your ego has no place on the mat.

It is very important that the teacher has control of the classroom; she needs to be able to speak-up when issues arise. For example, many yoga teachers tell students to listen to their own body while in class. This could mean resting instead of doing a posture, or adapting the posture for your own needs, or staying in the posture a shorter or longer period of time. Sometimes, however, there is a student who interprets this to mean he can do his own thing, like do a head stand while everyone else is in a supine position. This then becomes a safety issue.

The students lying next to him are in a very vulnerable position both physically and emotionally. What if he loses his balance and falls on them? So, you want a teacher who can set boundaries and rules and makes certain they are followed. Your physical safety is not the only area of wellbeing where you need to have a concern; emotional safety is equally important.

CHAPTER 4- PRACTICING YOGA-NOT JUST PHYSICAL SAFETY…

The practice of yoga often leads to emotional awareness and release. Sometimes, a pose can release emotional energy; it can be laughing, crying, or something in between - a feeling that is not definable, but present all the same. For many yoga students, that is the beauty of yoga; it enables the inner self to open and expand to the authentic self. Even if you never have an emotional release in a yoga class, you want to have a yoga teacher that honors and respects the student's process. The teacher should never berate, laugh at, judge, or criticize their students. While a teacher sometimes needs to correct a student, it is always done with respect and concern. Emotional safety also includes improper touching.

In many styles of yoga, the teacher will help the student with hands-on assists. Hands on assists done properly are yummy; they can make the posture go from feeling okay to giving the student an "aha" moment. They can help correct alignment issues, or help stretch a stubborn muscle. However, not everyone likes to be touched, and unfortunately, a few teachers have used assists to touch students improperly.

When initiating an assist, the teacher needs to ask before touching you and tell you where they are going to place their hands. If a teacher does touch you and you think it was improper, wait until the end of class and speak to them about it. Do not let it go unnoticed; give the teacher a chance to explain. It may have been accidental because a hand can brush one part of the body while adjusting another part. It could also have been a lack of communication, or a misunderstanding of cultural values between you and the teacher. It is better to clear the air, and tell them if you no longer want any hands-on assist.

After speaking to the teacher, if the touching continues and seems inappropriate, stop attending that class. In addition, if the teacher puts you on the defensive or does not take you seriously, do not go back. Also, notify the studio owner and if the teacher is registered notify the organization that holds their registration. Of course, if you ever think you were sexually assaulted by a teacher, report it to the police.

The other ethical safety issue for students with regards to their teacher is the relationship you have with them outside the classroom. Here are some things to consider: Yoga teachers do not enter into romantic relationships with their students. Because a yoga class can have the potential to be a sexually charged arena, it is up to the teacher to moderate the sexual energy and not give into it inside or outside the classroom.

Given the nature of many yoga classes, healthy friendships can develop. However, there is a fine line between the teacher and student when it comes to friendships. It is up to the teacher to make sure there is a teacher/student balance. If a teacher asks you out on a date, question his integrity and ethical standards.

Since yoga is a discipline where a person can delve into emotional issues, some students transfer their feelings to their teacher, much like a patient does to a psychologist, or a parishioner does to a minister. However, it is the teacher's responsibility to recognize this and to act accordingly. Along with your body and emotional safety, you will want to check out the safety of the classroom.

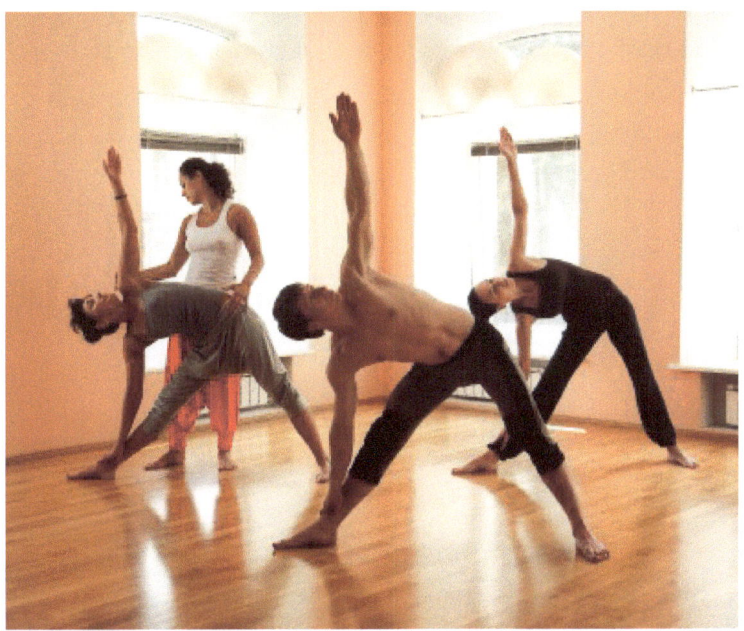

Condition of the Classroom

Take notice of the physical aspects of the building and the room where the classes are held. The room should be clean and neat. In the case of a fire, how would you get out of the building? If the teacher uses candles, is she mindful in placement of them? Does she leave the candles unattended? You want to make sure the floor is not slippery or that some sort of non-slip mat is required. Sometimes hands and feet can become sweaty while in a pose, so you want them on a surface that helps to prevent them from sliding. Sometimes no matter the surface, some hands will still sweat and slip. It will help if the teacher has towels or tissues, or bring your own. Access to a bathroom is important.

While most yoga styles use very little equipment, a few do, so you want to make sure the equipment is in good working order. Now that you are aware of safety concerns, your next step in having a satisfying yoga experience is choosing a style that is compatible with you. This can make a difference in how dedicated you become to yoga, or if you go back for a second experience.

CHAPTER 5- YOGA STYLES

The yoga of the ancients was not so much about the physical aspect of doing poses; it was about developing one's inner landscape or spirituality. However, when yoga came west it took on many transformations, resulting in many styles of yoga. One aspect that some schools of yoga have changed is the guru/student paradigm; a few styles no longer accept that an individual should be devoted to one teacher. Knowing what style of yoga is being taught, the dynamics of the organization, and what that tradition involves will make a huge difference in whether it jives with your expectations. It will also help you to get the most out of your yoga class.

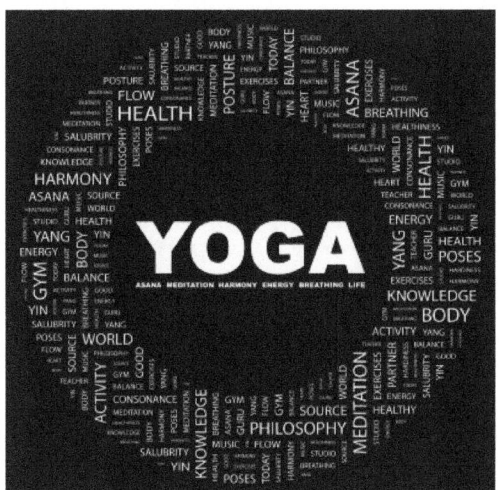

In the United States, the basis for most styles of yoga is hatha yoga. Hatha yoga is closely related to the raja yoga path that has 8 branches, which asanas (posture) is one of them. The asanas (postures) in hatha yoga are believed to be conduits between the body and a person's spirituality. In the U.S. the styles of hatha yoga varies, based more or less on the level of spirituality incorporated into the practice.

In addition, adherence to strict body alignment, regimented and vigorous posture flow, rooms with high temperatures and humidity, chanting, and the length that postures are held are some of the other differences in the schools of yoga. Before going to a class, research the style of yoga to see if it is something that interests you. Also, when you find a class you think you may want to attend, call the teacher and ask her to describe the type of yoga she teaches and what you can expect to do in the class.

With varying degrees and approaches, most yoga styles teach that yoga incorporates the three bodies, the physical body, the mental body, and the spiritual body. Be aware that because the word yoga is used in a title of a class, does not mean that it has much connection to the traditional practice of yoga. Some practices using the word yoga are, "water yoga," "hot nude yoga," "dog yoga," "sex yoga," or "dance yoga." This is why it is important that your expectations meet the reality of the class.

Yoga and Your Expectations

The last but not least thing to consider in choosing a yoga class is your expectations. What is it that you want right now from a yoga class? As you age or life situation changes, the style of yoga you want to practice may also change. Do not feel that you have to stick with one style or one certain teacher for your entire life. Tryout the different styles of yoga that interest you by taking a class or two in each one.

Most major types of yoga incorporate the yoga postures; you have to decide how much of it do you want. Where do you want the scale tipped? Are you looking for a spiritual awakening to yourself and the universe? Or do you want the focus to be on a good physical work-out, aspiring for the flexibility of a chimp? The spiritually pointed yoga will give at least as much time to the inner life as to the physical self. In the physically pointed yoga, the yoga is physically intense with less time on the inner life.

Sometimes finding the right yoga class match is like finding the right mate - it is about trial and error. You may have to try a few styles and teachers before you find your fit. However, the one place you do not want to gloss over is safety, both physical and emotional.

CHAPTER 6- HOW TO LOSE WEIGHT WITH BIKRAM YOGA

Bikram Yoga & Weight Loss

The combination of 100-degree heat and movement through the 26 postures of Bikram yoga can help you lose weight throughout your body. Although it's not possible to target your weight loss efforts only toward your belly, you will lose weight around your midsection as your overall weight decreases. According to the Mayo Clinic, regular yoga practice can help you make better and healthier lifestyle habits that contribute toward further weight loss and an increase in your overall well-being.

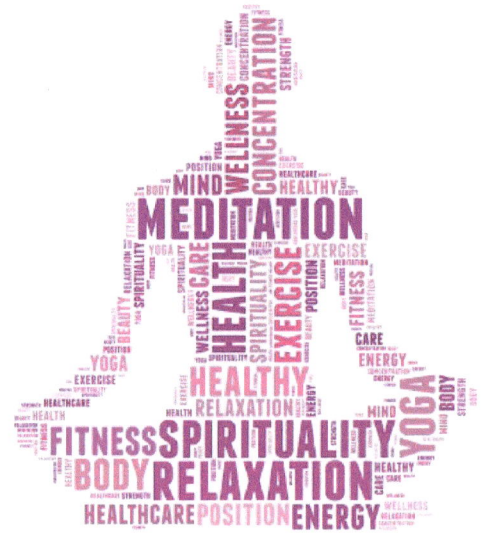

A Healthy Lifestyle

Practicing Bikram yoga regularly is an excellent part of an overall healthy lifestyle plan. To make the time spent on yoga effective, it's important to eat a healthy diet that helps to fuel your body. Since Bikram yoga helps calm the body and mind, you'll also enjoy reduced stress and a relaxing peacefulness in your mind and body, according to the Mayo Clinic.

Gaining Strength & Muscle

Many of the 26 postures used in Bikram yoga are weight-bearing exercises. These postures help your muscles to become stronger, and they help you develop lean muscle mass. Muscle weighs more than fat, so as you lose fat and develop more muscle, the numbers on the weight scale might not change very much. But leaner, toned muscles will give you a thinner appearance all over your body, including your belly area. Lean muscle also burns calories more efficiently than fat, which can contribute toward the loss of fat in your belly and throughout your body.

A Toned Midsection

Toned muscles in the abdominal area can play a huge role in the appearance of your belly. As you lose weight by practicing Bikram yoga and engaging in aerobic exercise, such as walking or biking, the muscles of your midsection will also become tighter and more toned. These tight, toned muscles act as a natural girdle to make your midsection look more physically fit.

CHAPTER 7- 26 POSTURES USED IN BIKRAM YOGA

First Breathing Exercise

Standing Deep Breathing- Pranayama (Sanskrit)

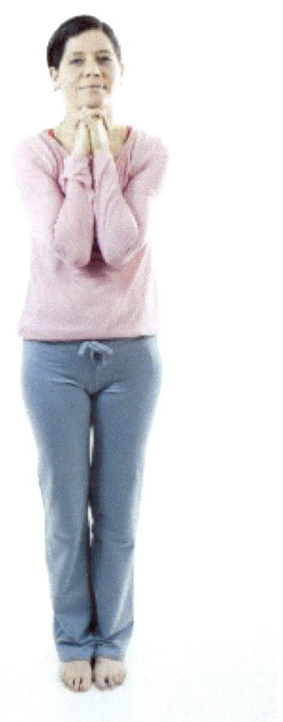

Posture 1

Half Moon Pose-Ardha-Chandrasana (Sanskrit)

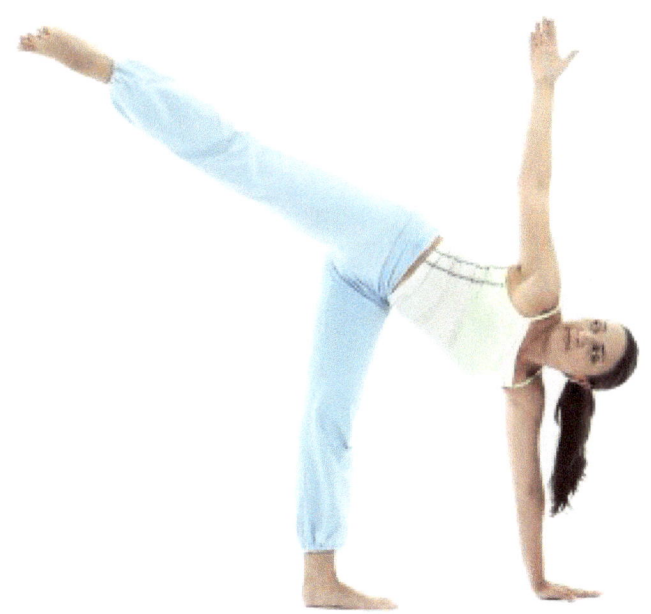

Posture 2

Hands To Feet Pose-Pada-Hastasana

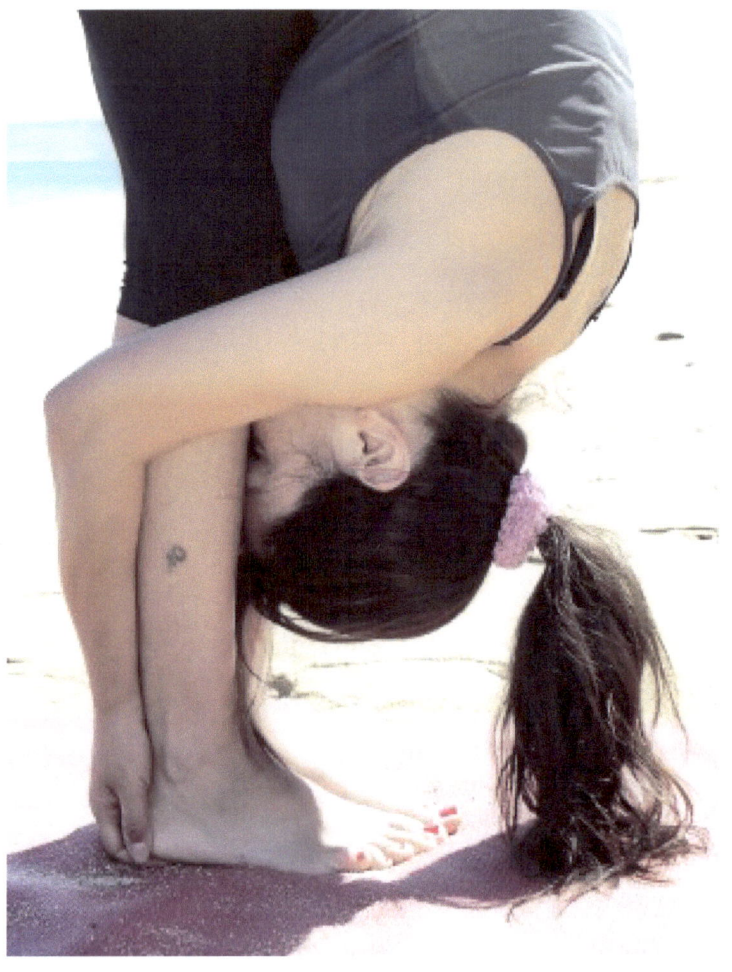

Posture 3

Awkward Pose- Utkatasana (Sanskrit)

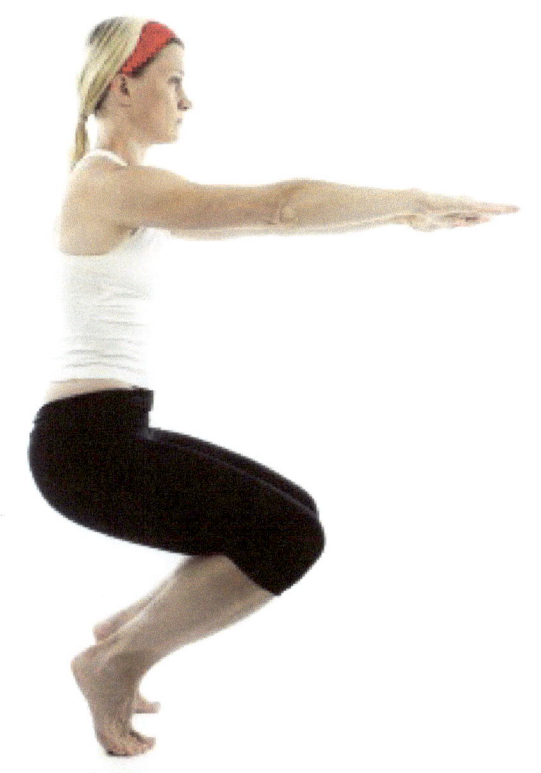

Posture 4

Eagle Pose- Garurasana (Sanskrit)

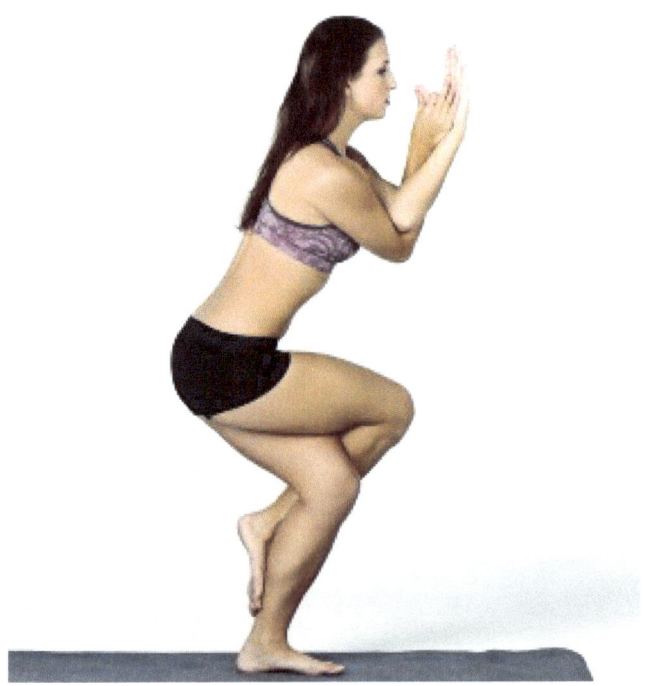

Posture 5

Standing Head to Knee- Dandayamana-Janushirasana
(Sanskrit)

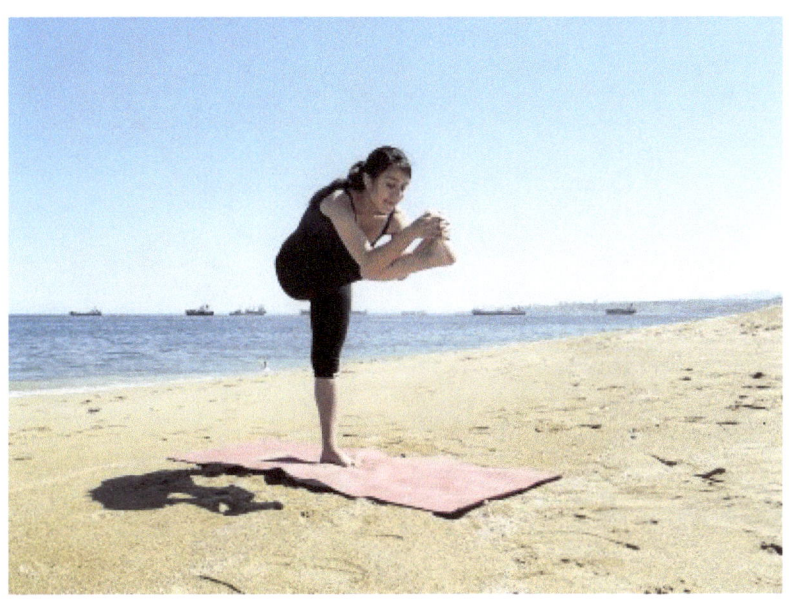

Posture 6

Standing Bow Pulling Pose - Dandayamana-Dhanurasana
(Sanskrit)

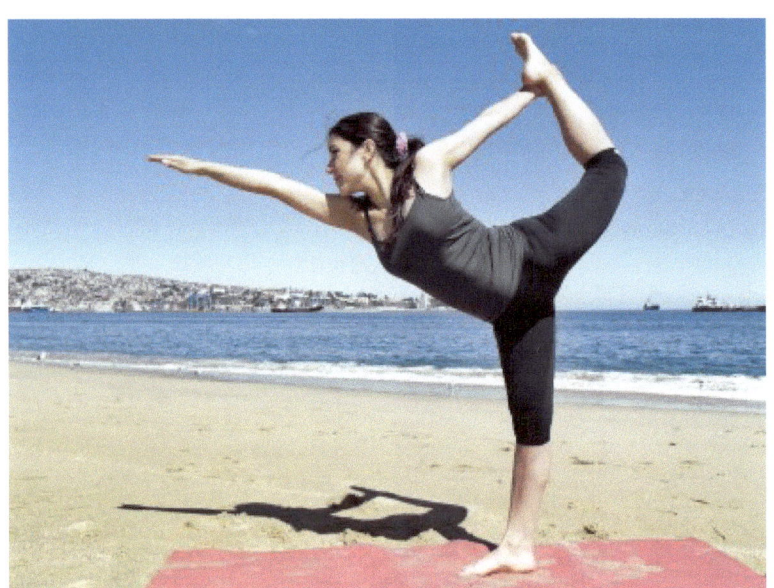

Posture 7

Balancing Stick- Tuladandasana (Sanskrit)

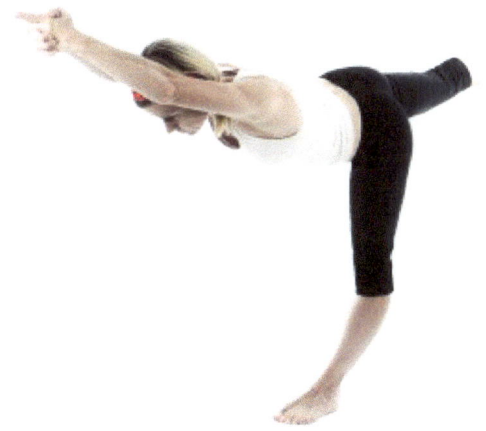

Posture 8

Standing Separate Leg Stretching Pose- Dandayamana-
Bibhaktapada-Paschimotthanasana (Sanskrit)

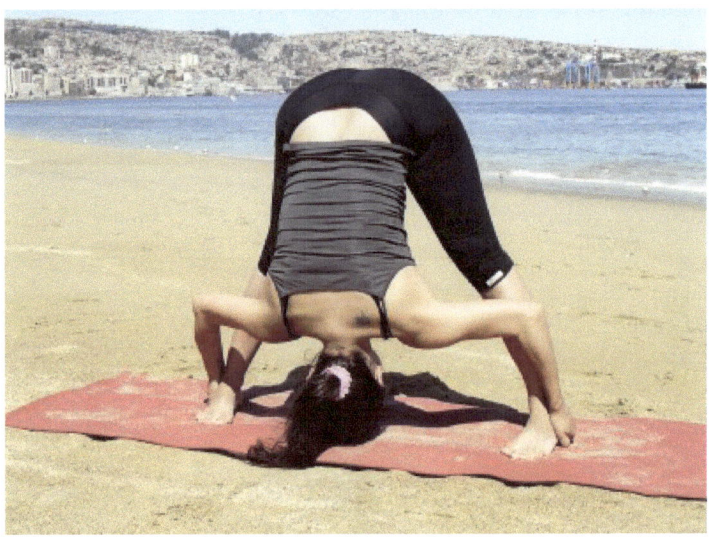

Posture 9

Triangle Pose- Trikanasana (Sanskrit)

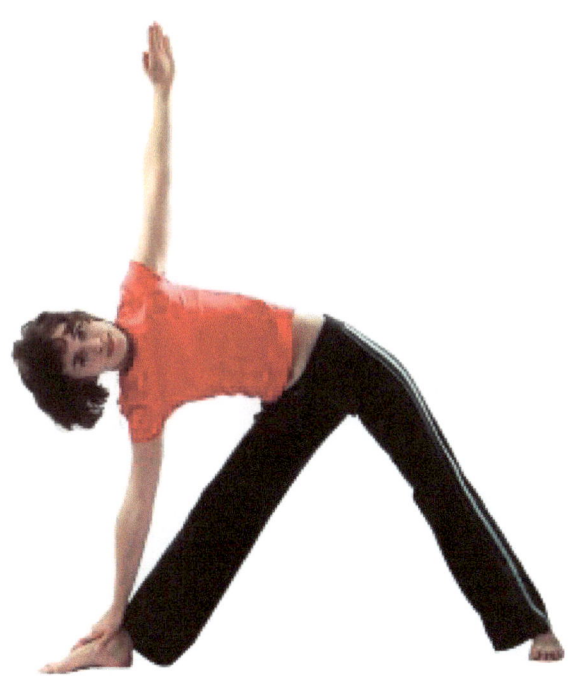

Posture 10

Standing Separate Leg Head to Knee Pose- Dandayamana-
Bibhaktapada-Janushirasana (Sanskrit)

Posture 11

Tree Pose- Tadasana (Sanskrit)

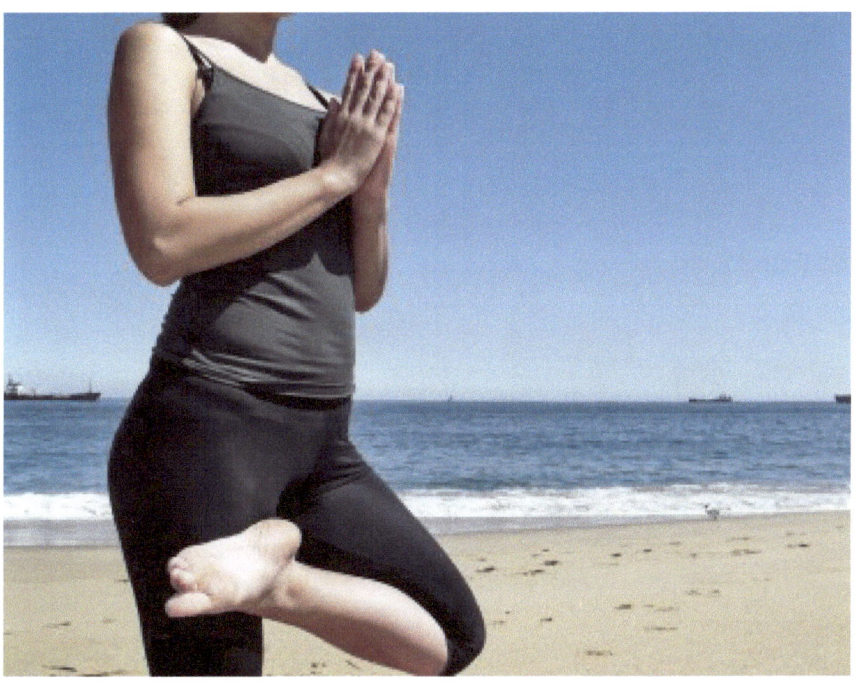

Posture 12

Toe Stand-Padangustasana (Sanskrit)

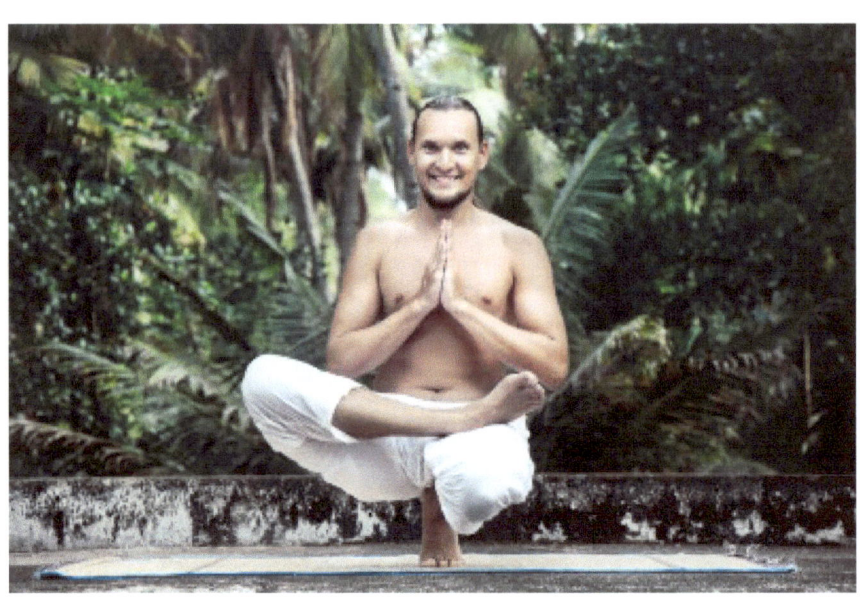

Posture 13

Dead Body Pose- Savasana(Sanskrit)

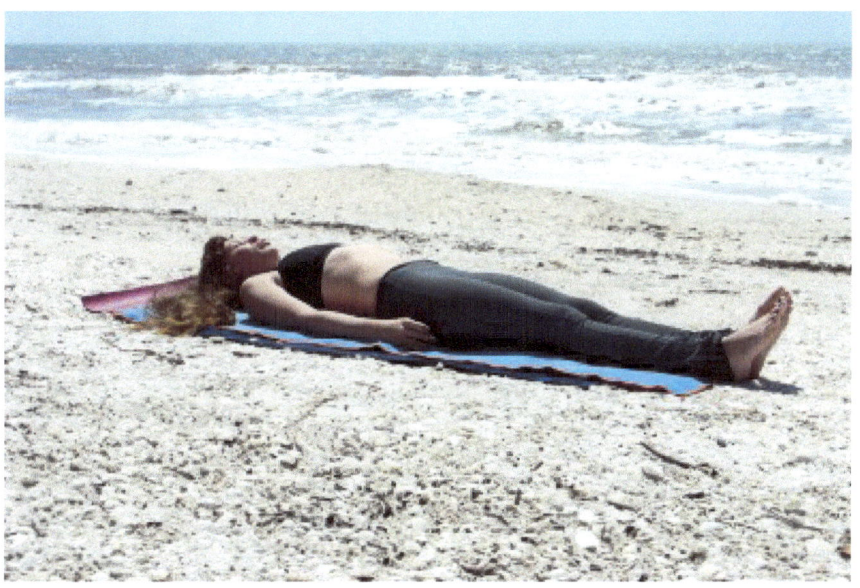

Posture 14

Wind-Removing Pose- Pavanamuktasana(Sanskrit)

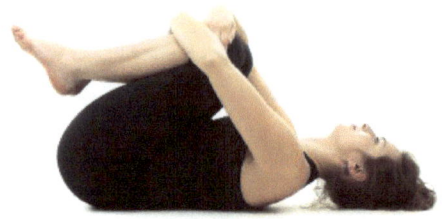

Sit up- Pada-Hasthasana (Sanskrit)

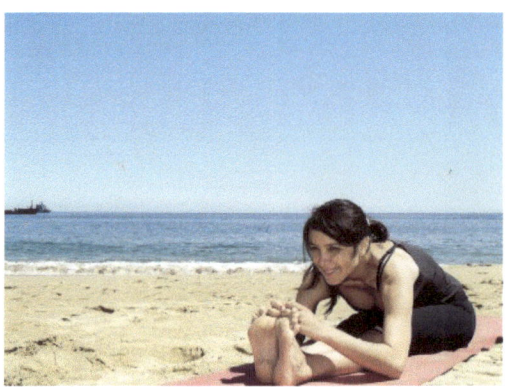

Posture 15

Cobra Pose- Bhujangasana (Sanskrit)

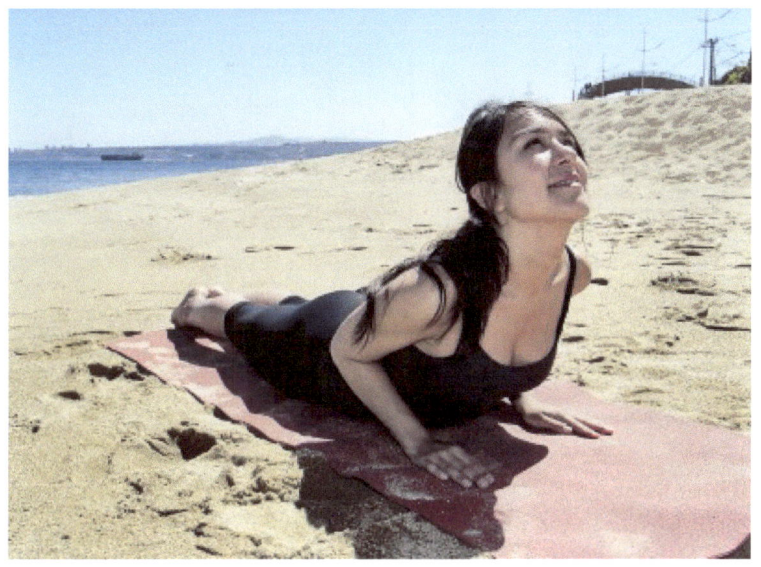

Posture 16

Locust Pose-Salabhasana (Sanskrit)

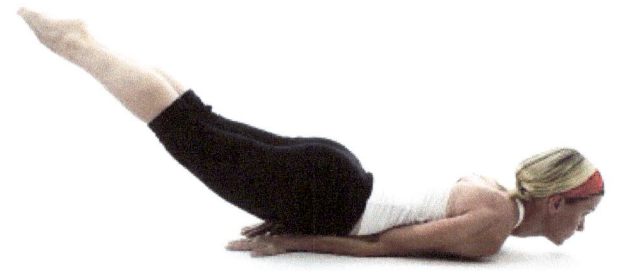

Posture 17

Full Locust Pose-Poorna-Salabhasana (Sanskrit)

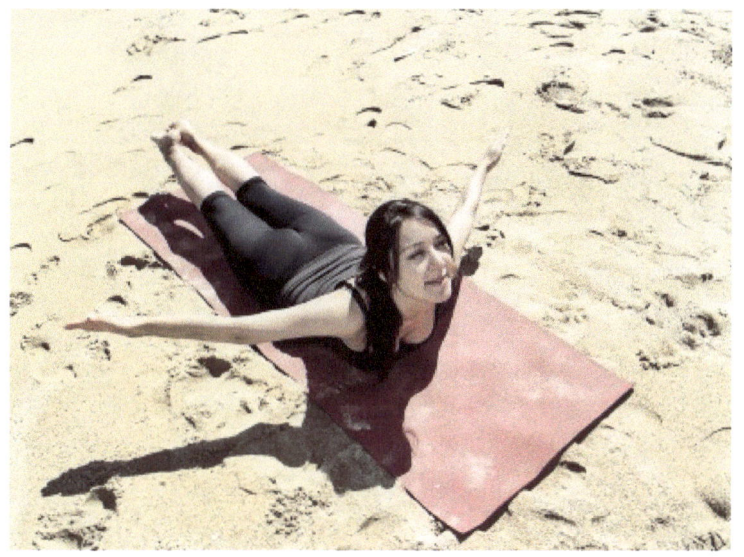

Posture 18

Bow Pose-Dhanurasana (Sanskrit)

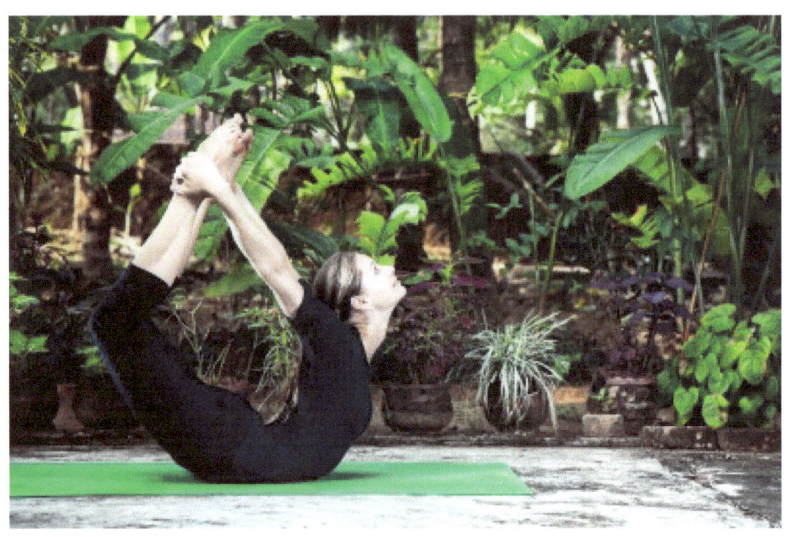

Posture 19

Fixed Firm Pose- Supta-Vajrasana (Sanskrit)

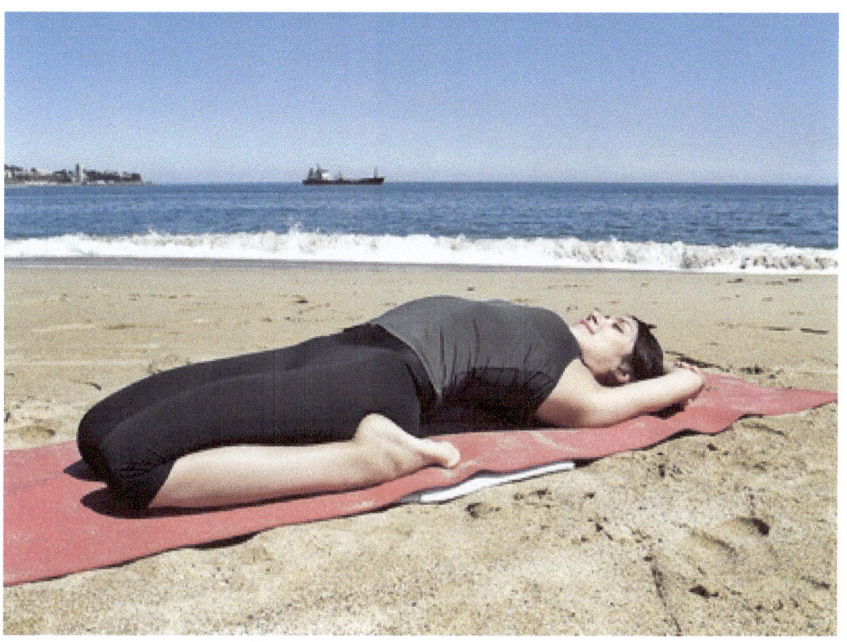

Posture 20

Half Tortoise Pose- Ardha-Kurmasana(Sanskrit)

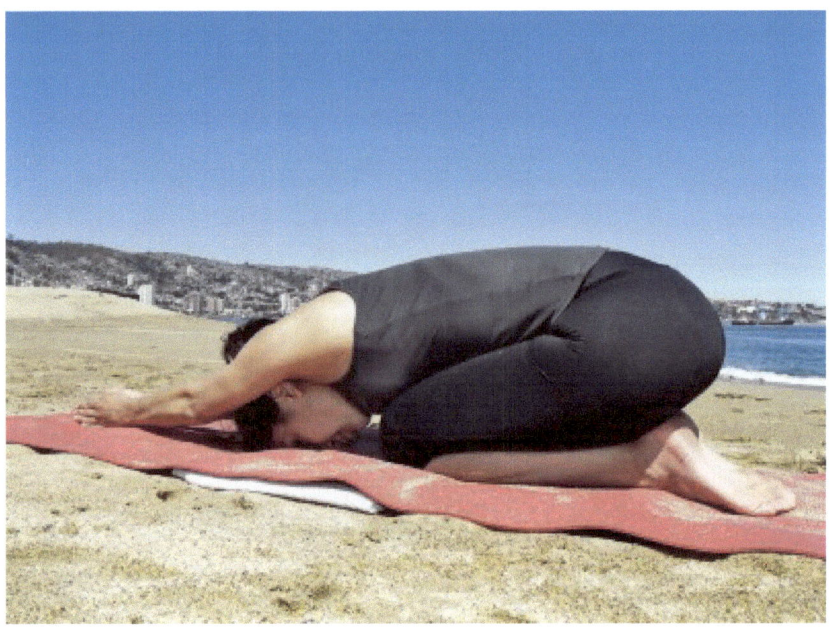

Posture 21

Camel Pose- Ustrasana (Sanskrit)

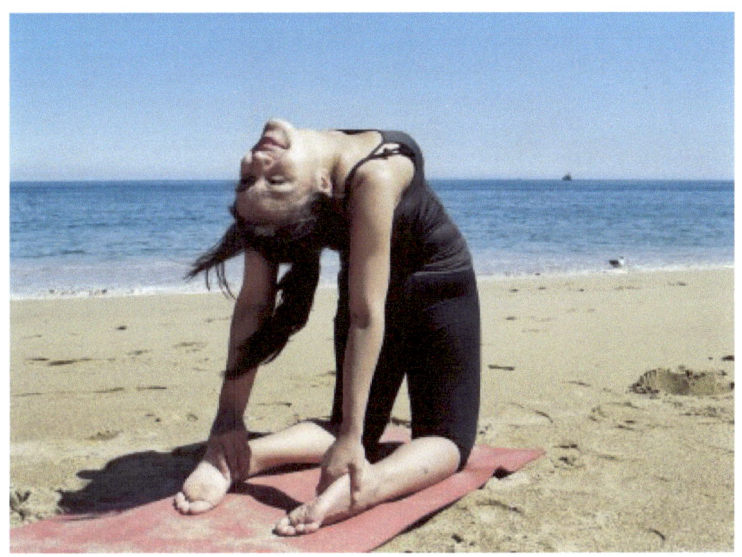

Posture 22

Rabbit Pose- Sasangasana (Sanskrit)

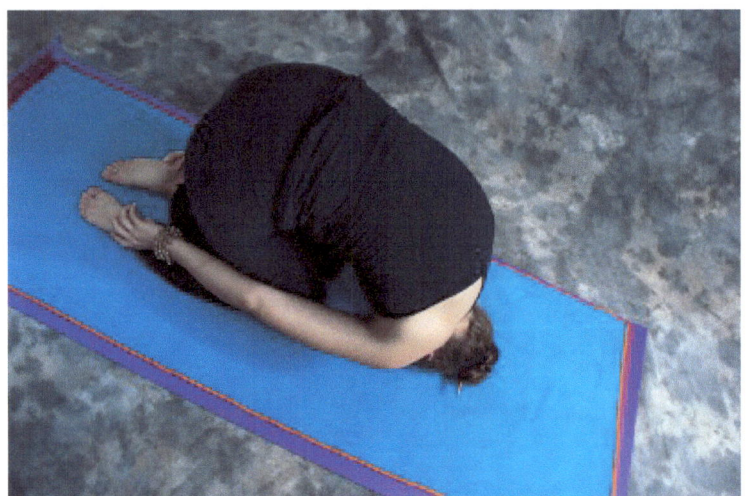

Posture 23 & 24

Head to Knee Pose and Stretching Pose-Janushirasana and
Paschimotthanasana (Sanskrit)

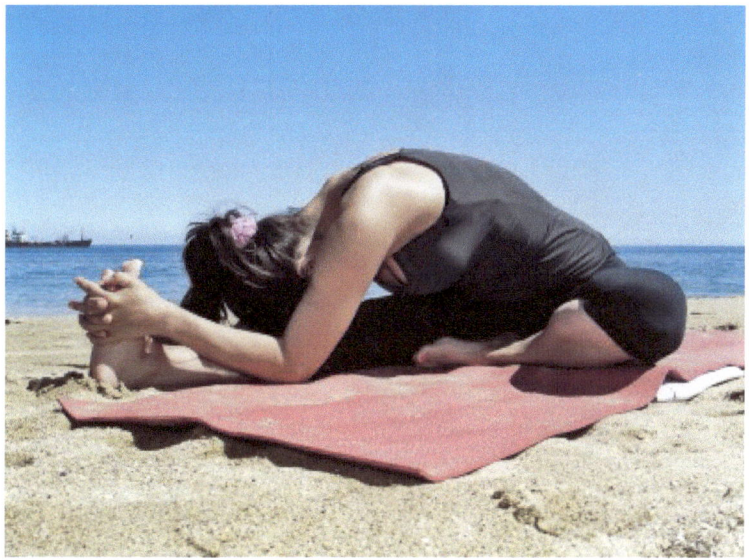

Posture 25

Spine-Twisting Pose- Ardha-Matsyendrasana (Sanskrit)

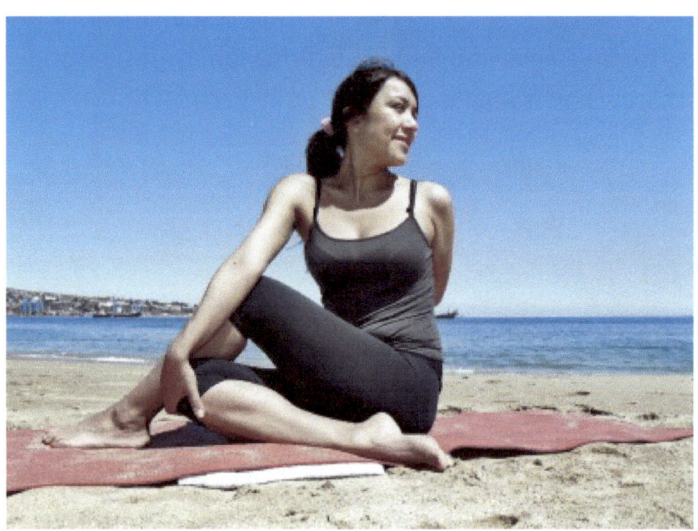

2nd Breathing Exercise & Posture 26

Blowing in Firm Pose- Kapalbhati in
Vajrasana(Sanskrit)

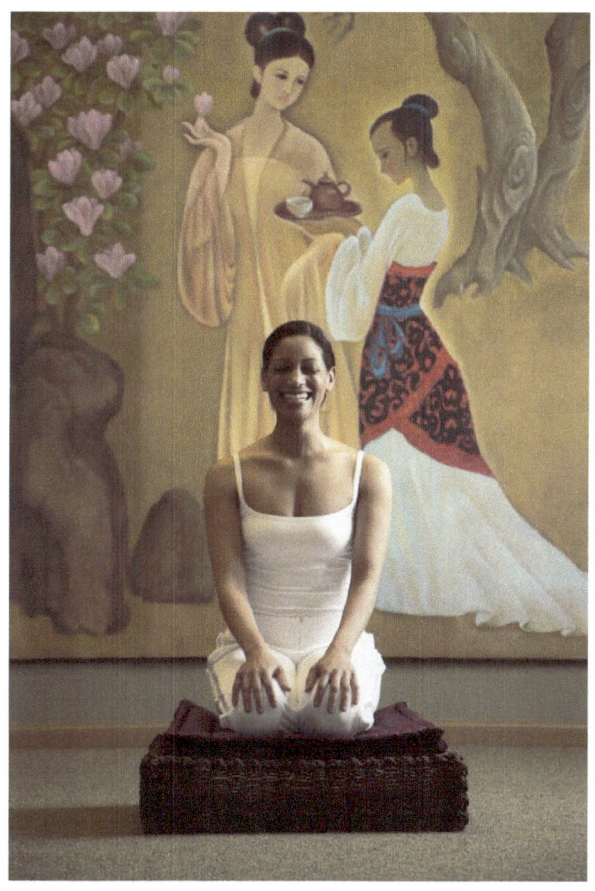

CHAPTER 8- MOKSHA: A NEW KIND OF HOT YOGA

Another form of hot yoga known as Moksha yoga was started in 2004 by Jessica Robertson and Ted Grand in Toronto, Canada. It is one of the new forms of yoga on the block and has quickly worked its way into many yoga studios all over the world. The yoga poses (approximately 40) are done in a hot room (similar to Bikram yoga). The studios that practice this form of yoga also have to adhere to a specific set of rules that require that the spaces are environmentally friendly and that natural cleansers and building materials are used.

How to Locate a Moksha Studio

The studios where one can practice Moksha are owned by yoga teachers that are approved by the founders Jessica Robertson and Ted Grant. There are many yoga studios that have the name Moksha as when translated it means enlightenment or freedom so you have to do your checks and balances before going to a session.

An Overview of the Experience

Moksha yoga starts out with Savasana and ends with it as well. On numerous occasions persons participating in the yoga session have to set the intention before they start to do the standing poses. After executing the standing poses, the session moves on to floor sequences that include spinal work, upper body work and hip openers. This form of yoga helps to prolong health and can be challenging.

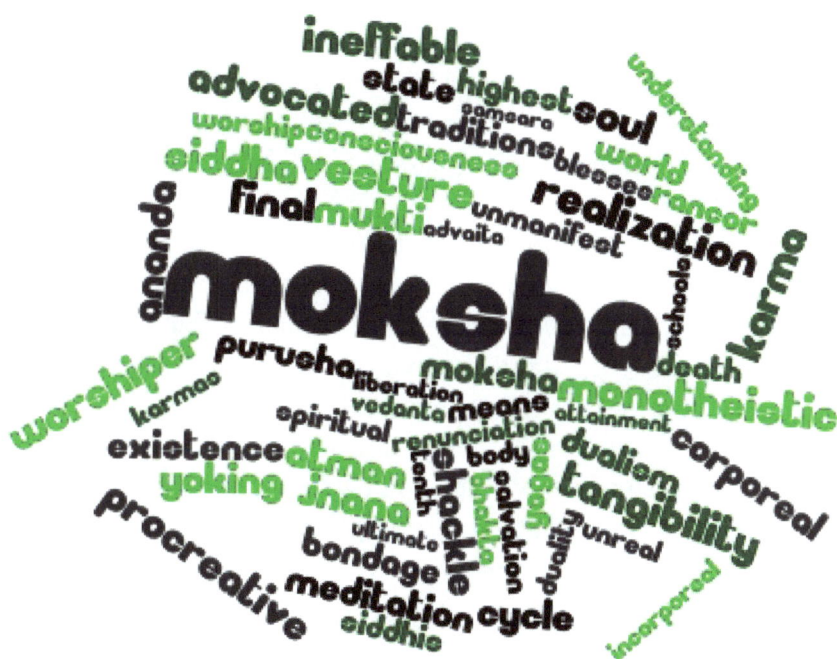

Bikram and Moksha Hot Yoga- The Subtle Differences

An Overview of Bikram Hot Yoga

A native of India, Bikram Choudhury is the creator of this form of yoga and he started this form of yoga along with his wife in Beverly Hills. The style of yoga was named after him.

An Overview of Moksha Hot Yoga

This form of hot yoga was started by Jessica Robertson and Ted Grand in 2004. They are based in Toronto. This form of yoga focuses mainly on social consciousness and this is reflected through karma classes (where students can pay what they can afford), studios that are environmentally friendly and community initiatives.

Based on information placed on the Moksha website they state that they are a set of autonomous yoga studios that are founded on living that is environmentally conscious, ethical and compassionate. It is also believed that yoga is accessible to all.

The studios tend to be fitted with bamboo studio floors, cleaning products that are environmentally friendly, filtered faucets, heat panels that are energy efficient and use paints that are VOC free.

The Temperature in the Room

Based on information placed on the Bikram website, the studio has to be at a temperature between 104 and 105 degrees Fahrenheit. The Moksha studios are at the same temperature as well.

The question that many may ask is why the studio has to be so hot. From a theoretical perspective, practicing yoga in a room that is hot will allow the joints and muscles in the body to stretch and soften and then the individual will be better able to ha e more full range of motion.

The Yoga Poses

There is a slight difference between the number of poses in Bikram yoga and Moksha yoga. Bikram has twenty six poses while Moksha has forty. A lot of the poses are similar but it appears that more variation is in the Moksha poses.

As it relates to the Moksha classes- there is not one single class for this form of yoga. There is Ashtanga, Vinyasa and other classes that are offered.

In terms of the sequence that the class follows it starts out with a corpse pose (svasana) and is followed by standing poses which then transition to floor poses and end with another savasana. Moksha yoga also has a number of flows vinyasa (downward dog) flows while Bikram yoga has none.

As it relates to Bikram classes- there are twenty six yoga poses that are done in the same sequence in each class. The instructor makes no changes to the routine.

The Class Setting

One of the most noticeable differences between Moksha and Bikram yoga is the way that the instructions are delivered. As mentioned beforehand the Bikram classes have no form of variation as everything is scripted. The instructor remains on a platform and delivers the instructions. There is constant yoga chatter which is said to keep the level of focus intact and prevent minds from wandering.

On the other hand Moksha has no shouted instructions and there can be variation in the way the classes are instructed.

Other differences between Moksha Hot Yoga and Bikram Hot Yoga

Bikram is a bit more demanding and intimidating than Moksha yoga. The latter has an instructor that speaks more gently and slowly and the students can work on getting as close to the pose as they can without being pressured to get it right from the outset.

In a Bikram yoga class the students are always reminded that the poses require their full dedication.

Length of the Class

Bikram is set at an hour and thirty minutes for each class while Moksha can run from an hour to one hour and thirty minutes.

The Advantages of Moksha and Bikram Hot Yoga

Triggers weight loss

Helps relieve the symptoms of asthma, insomnia, muscular pain, arthritis and stress

Promotes detoxification

Improves mental clarity

Better flexibility

Better psychological and physical well being

Muscles that are tones and strong

Which Form of Hot Yoga is Better?

That is pretty much up to the individual to decide. I personally found Bikram yoga to be much more physically and mentally demanding than Moksha. Moksha tends to be much more calming and peaceful and gives the same results in the long run. Moksha also has variation which some may prefer as opposed to doing the same set of poses in the same way at each session.

A lot of us never take a deep breath for the entire day. The most common practice in yoga is to take a deep breath through the nose. This intake of breath ought to pull the diaphragm down as the lungs fill up. If you observe a child sleeping you will see the stomach rising and falling. This is the same action that adults should be doing. On the matter of exhalation, work on sucking the belly button in and imagine it touching the spine. This action will push up the diaphragm and all the air will then be expelled from the lungs. When this is done more nitric oxide will be sent to the lungs and put more oxygen in the body.

The practice of yoga will help to rid the body of any buildup of waste. This is done through a process called lymphatic simulation. Yoga helps to loosen joints and muscles that typically do not get used during daily activities. There are a number of routines that help increase the flow of blood through the body like sun salutation. Through yoga and individual also learns how to handle the weight of the body and also helps to make the body less susceptible to damage as it improves muscle strength and build bone.

The practice of yoga helps the individual to place more focus on certain parts of the body such as the tight joints and muscles. Bear in mind that yoga can prove difficult in the initial stages for someone who has a problem focusing the mind. After a while of practice, it will become much easier to focus.

Contrary to what many believe, the practice of yoga is much more than a physical exercise. It is the path to a new way of life that focuses on both the outer and inner realities. One can always read up on the various forms of yoga but you will never truly understand it unless you practice it.

The practice of yoga is a way of life and the newest forms of yoga, Bikram and Moksha hot yoga are just new ways in which the individual can have an experience that will affect both the body and the mind. It cannot be mentioned enough that the practice of yoga is an experience which is what makes it unique from any other form of exercise. The body not gets a great workout and the mind gets reset.

This is why it is recommended that yoga be practiced early in the mornings and in the evenings after work. You can get the mind and body ready to face the day and in the evening you can get rid of all the negative energy and stress that was accumulated throughout the course of the day.

ABOUT THE AUTHOR

Amy Gilchrist has been a student of the traditional forms of yoga for many years and then started to do research on the hot forms of yoga as they started to become more popular. She was intrigued by the fact that these forms of yoga were carried out in rooms set to a certain temperature. Not one to balk at a challenge she took it upon herself to try out both forms to see if she would add this to the growing list of yoga styles that she was on her way to mastering.

Not one to go on a journey without sharing, she made the decision to document everything that she had experienced and to use some of that information to write a book that would help others to have an understanding of the two forms of hot yoga as well. Amy provides wonderful insight into the world of Bikram and Moksha hot yoga.